Stroke of God

A STROKE SURVIVORS JOURNEY

LOUIS TURBEVILLE

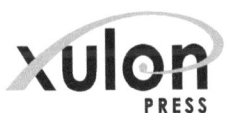

Copyright © 2015 by Louis Turbeville

Stroke of God
A stroke survivors journey
by Louis Turbeville

Printed in the United States of America.

ISBN 9781498434775

All rights reserved solely by the author. The author guarantees all contents are original and do not infringe upon the legal rights of any other person or work. No part of this book may be reproduced in any form without the permission of the author. The views expressed in this book are not necessarily those of the publisher.

Unless otherwise indicated, Scripture quotations taken from the New International Version (NIV). Copyright © 1973, 1978, 1984, 2011 by Biblica, Inc.™. Used by permission. All rights reserved.

www.xulonpress.com

Dedication

This book is first dedicated to three people who were my rocks through this journey. Without any of the three, combined with God's grace, I would not be where I am today. First to my doctor Abraham Thomas, you are an incredible gift to your profession. Your kindness, in the way you treated me, was unsurpassed by any other doctor I've ever come in contact with. Your understanding, your patience, and your reassurance that you AND God, would help me get through this gave me reason to believe. Next to Priya Das, my speech therapist at Memorial Hermann Southwest rehab, you were my guardian angel. You were blessed, by God, to do what you do. Your ability to reassure, when no one else could, kept me going. You, my dear, gave me reason to believe that SOMEONE, truly understood what my pea brain was feeling, what my fears were, and what my true needs were. You kept me going and got me through things that no one else understood. And for that, not even a thank you can repay. Last, but far from least, to my wife Cyndi, my soul mate and my eternal nurse in shining armor. You were amazingly brave and supported me like no other. You went beyond the call of duty. You were my advocate, like no other. You saved my life. I love you, my dearest, and hope I can be half the person to you as you are a hero to me. I love you.

There were others in this journey. I can't mention you all. But know this, all of you that stood by my side, held my hand, gave me a hug, and especially those that prayed for me, I thank you. I hope someday I can return the favor. My start to that is to write this book. The whole reason for the book is to possibly give back just a little of what each of you gave to me, and to give someone, maybe not as lucky as me, a little hope. A little hope. Helping someone say,"I'm going to be ok."

Acknowledgements

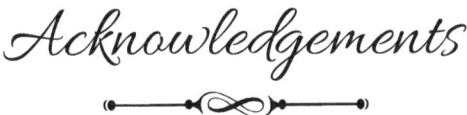

Life is so much like my favorite past-time – Baseball

Curves are part of playing the game.

We are told they exist.

We are told they are coming.

But until you are thrown that one nasty pitch

The one that breaks

That makes you duck

That makes you jump out of your skin

That makes you say

"what was that ?"

We never believe.

On a cold November day

I got thrown the curve ball of my life

The hook

The Hanger

The Breaker

The pitch that can make you go to your knees

Behind me was a team that would not allow me to quit

My sister Linda

My boys

My church Family

Nurses

Westin, Jaxon, Layton, Gordon

Therapists

Friends

James Johnson

Lori & Christine

So many touched and encouraged me when I needed you most.

Most of all, I learned my God was there for me.

He listened and answered prayers

He encouraged me

I thank my God for many more chances

Than I've ever deserved

Table of Contents

Introduction . . . . *xi*

Round 1 – The Heart *17*

Round 2 – Left Brain *29*

Round 3 – Right Brain. *45*

Round 4 – Recovery *59*

Reflection. *81*

Introduction

I know some will question my chosen title of this book, "Stroke of God", so I'll partially explain here in the beginning. First, the term "Stroke" was taken from a medical phrase coined in the 16th century "stroke from the hand of God." Blood clots and other brain maladies were a mystery that could only be explained as something coming from the hand of God. As I've reflected on my journey over the last year, the one thing I wanted to convey, was my appreciation of God's mercy through this ordeal. I have crossed paths with individuals that have questioned God and his purpose of inflicting such maladies such as Stroke, Heart disease, Cancer etc on us. How could a loving God do this to us? How could he do this to our loved ones? Why me?

Why my son, or wife? Probably a natural reaction by those who misunderstand God and his purpose. Although I'll agree with you, that God created everyone and everything, which includes the dreaded diseases above and many others, I won't agree that God points a finger at you or me and says "you're going to have this stroke, or whatever." God does allow these things to exist, and he does allow for bad things to happen to good people. But within all of those situations, there's room for God's grace on us. There is opportunity for all of us to use the situations that God allows, to glorify him. To use those small blessings, within tragedy, to glorify him. Why would we want to do that, when He's done this to us you say? Because of grace. Grace, is the good God has given us, namely Eternal life. One thing I've held on to during this journey, is that God's hand did touch me during this. Not to cripple or maim, but to heal. To bless me with mercy. To let me live on. To take something from him, and hopefully to give it to someone else.

This is a story of a normal 54 year old guy who thought he was fairly fit (kidding himself maybe?) A guy who biked, climbed mountains (small ones), played flag football and swam. I was a

Introduction

basic, active grandpa who thought he was 20 years younger than he actually was.

My Christian beliefs were very strong. And I'll say right now, God was with me the last year, no matter how bad things got or how serious things became. I have no doubt he was by my side. During my recovery I realized how lucky I was considering I was a person who had suffered a blocked artery and two strokes. I'm undoubtedly blessed to be sitting here typing this journey. God carried me through this. In the end it became evident to me that God had things he wanted me to do. Was it this book? I'm not sure at this point, but hopefully I can stay focused on him, and take this journey wherever he wants it to go.

> **He makes me lie down in green pastures, he leads me beside quiet waters, (Psalm 23:2 NIV)**

Although, in relative terms, my strokes may have been far less debilitating than yours, or possibly your loved ones, there was a newly gained perspective of stroke survivors and their families. I've now seen a stroke from the brain looking out, which taught me so much about what a stroke victim goes through. Maybe I don't understand it all, considering the level of stroke I had, but I now understand so much, I feel compelled to try and convey, especially to family members of stroke victims, a little understanding of what we see and feel. Hopefully, your learned insight will help support your loved one.

The Lord is good to all; he has compassion on all he has made. (Psalm 145:9 NIV)

It's funny how God works things out too. As I set out on this journey to write this story, I suddenly went from the stoke survivor, to the support role. As I'm writing this I sit by my wife Cyndi's' bedside at the hospital. She was diagnosed with a blood clot to her kidney in the last few days, and has lost 10% of her kidney function. Certainly not a stroke, but in some ways similar. Instead of a mystery blood clot traveling to the brain and depriving the brain of precious oxygen, hers deprived her kidney. Now the rock of my life, the earthly great supporter who carried me through, is walking in my shoes. Unexpected? Out of the blue? A loved one struck by one of the great mysteries of the body. So many unanswered questions. Not only by the patient, but by the ones who love and surround them.

> *As for me, this mystery has been revealed to me, not because I have greater wisdom than anyone else alive, but so that Your Majesty may know the interpretation and that you may understand what went through your mind. (Daniel 2:30 NIV)*

Round 1

The Heart

This journey for me started very subtle. Early 2013, I started having what I thought was acid reflux. Occasionally, heartburn would arise, which I tried self-medicating with medicines I had been given in the past, for reflux. Although it seemed to help, the symptoms seemed to get more and more intense and more frequent as the months went by. On a short vacation to Port Lavaca, suddenly the symptoms became unbearable. Every meal was accompanied by intense pain in my chest as I ate. Each swallow was followed by pain of the food going down my esophagus to my stomach. I could feel every bite as it traveled down into my stomach. Monday morning, I called my gastrointestinal doctor and got an appointment for that day. A quick office visit turned into a trip to the pharmacy to prep for an endoscopy (throat) and an colonoscopy for the next day.

Both tests were ones Cyndi and I were very familiar with. Each of us had our share of each over the years, due to IBS, diverticulitis, and polyps. Dr Haddad, informed us he had removed several pre-cancerous polyps and my esophagus was inflamed, probably due to the acid reflux. Dexilant was prescribed for the acid and we went on our way.

> **Finally, brothers and sisters, whatever is true, whatever is noble, whatever is right, whatever is pure, whatever is lovely, whatever is admirable—if anything is excellent or praiseworthy—think about such things. (Philippians 4:8 NIV)**

Several weeks went by with the pain coming and going. Never, ever was the pain associated with exertion, only when eating. Odd thing learned from this, the medical text books are far from complete. The pain I experienced was not anywhere typical for the diagnoses I would shortly receive. Three weeks after starting the Dexilant, I marched back to the Dr Haddad for a follow-up. Because Gastro doctors are typically very busy people, it's very common, at least in our experience, to deal with PA's. This is very aggravating to me at times, because I always felt I was getting the "second team" and not the expert. In this case, this PA would make a diagnoses maybe some would call a lucky guess or a hunch that would literally save my life. Dr. Blaise looked at me and suggested that I go have some test run just to eliminate other possibilities. She wanted me to go directly to the ER of the hospital across the street to have an EKG, and an enzyme study run to eliminate a heart issue. I'll have to say, I left that doctors office thinking, she's off her rocker. I'm a healthy guy. I had no blood pressure issues. My cholesterol numbers were decent, and this is insane. I got in my car, headed home, calling Cyndi and told her what a crazy idea this PA had wanting me to go to the ER to sit there for hours for this nonsense testing. Thank God Cyndi talked sense into me and convinced me that maybe, just maybe, it would be a good idea to eliminate this as a problem. So, at 5:00 on a Monday afternoon, I turned my truck around and headed to the ER of Patients Hospital.

Moses answered the people, "Do not be afraid. Stand firm and you will see the deliverance the Lord will bring you today. (Exodus 14:13 NIV)

So in I walked. Steadily asking myself, "Why am I here?" I explained to the nurse the issues, and they quickly took me back to triage me. Blood pressure, heart rate, temp, and EKG were all normal. No heart attack. Blood was drawn for enzyme study. Nitro glycerin patch was put on my chest. An IV was placed in my arm. Go sit in the waiting room. Here's the waiting part… 1,2,3,4 hours go by. Finally get called back. "We have a stretcher for you." 11:30, cardiologist comes in, goes over history, tells me "I don't think anything wrong with your heart, but let's go ahead and run these test while we have you here". "See! Even he says this is silly", I say to Cyndi. But we're here, let's finish what we started. 1,2,3,4 more hours go by. Finally, they decide they want to keep me and transfer me to a room. 11 hours after walking in ER, I'm finally in a room with a real bed.

Fast forward to later that day (Tuesday), Cardiologist came back around and discusses ideas and options. Main plan of action…a stress test. At that time I question him on if he'd do a nuclear test or not. He told me "normally no," but we could if I really wanted. I stated "Yes I want a full nuclear test" especially if we we're going to go through the trouble. I had already been coached by my RN sister, Linda, that the nuclear test was much more accurate. The Cardiologist again stressed to me, he didn't feel they would find anything wrong.

Wednesday rolls around. Wait, wait, wait. Nurse comes in around 2:00 to give me an injection for nuclear portion of test. Later, I read that the substance injected is Thallium. A substance in some form used in rat poison. Nice, huh? Never the less, in today's form, it enables testing similar to a CAT scan that shows blood flow through our arteries during a stress test. As the stress test starts, the cardiologist again re-assures me that he expects to find nothing, and plans on discharging me that evening, and that I should follow-up with him in a week. Stress test goes as I expected. I get on treadmill, start running, and target 140 beats per min. Just as I hit the target the doctor abruptly stops the test and tells the tech he's seen enough. Then he walks out of the room. All the wires are detached, another nuclear scan is done, and I'm wheeled back to my room. By 4:00 or 4:30, I'm back in my room fully expecting to be discharged. Never happens. Not a word. Another night in the hospital, and don't I even know why.

Thursday morning comes, and the cardiologist strolls in about 10:00. He abruptly informs me that he saw some irregularities during the stress test. He wants to do further testing to make sure there is not a problem. He informs me he has scheduled an angioplasty for that afternoon. Crushing news for me. I'm emotionally blown away. I'm already in my fourth day in the hospital having thought, and having been told, that there was most likely nothing wrong. Now on day four, I'm about to be wheeled into surgery to have a catheter stuck in my groin, to look at my heart and arteries. If anything is found, they will place a stent in to repair, OR, they will come out to discuss other options (i.e.... surgery). Devastation! Fear sets in! My mind takes over, and I become an emotional wreck.

It's funny, when we actually face the possibility of death, how differently we act as opposed to how we think we would act. Maybe that changes with age. Maybe when I'm 88, as opposed to 54, I'll look at death differently.

Two days ago, my sister called to inform me that my mother (88 years of age), who has been in a nursing home for 4 years, is sick with pneumonia and is refusing treatment. Hospice is being called in to make her comfortable, this is something Cyndi and I are very familiar with. Cyndi's mom spent her last year in our home under Hospice care. Definition of Hospice–waiting... Mom is tired of fighting, living, and existing. That's ok, I guess. I hope when the time comes, I'm ready to accept death. I guess that's the difference in a 54 year old and an 88 year old. I'm comfortable with my relationship with my God, but still feel I have things to do here on earth. At 88, I guess the gas just runs out, and we get to the point of not wanting to even take the short drives around the block anymore.

The saving grace of the day is I go for a walk, and I go to see Jimmy Reynolds. Jimmy is a good friend from church. Jimmy had just had surgery to remove a tumor and happened to be on the same floor as I was. As I walk in his room, J.D.Heim, another friend from church is sitting there visiting. After explaining what was going on, J.D. tells me he's had more than one angioplasty, and they were absolutely no big deal. I can't convey how reassuring this was to me, and thank God that J.D. was in that room that day. The fear is not gone, but the complete unknown that the doctor didn't have the sense to explain to me has been explained by a good man. You weren't there just to comfort Jimmy that day J.D., God had you there to comfort another.

A friend loves at all times, and a brother is born for a time of adversity. (Proverbs 17:17 NIV)

3:00 rolls around, and a nurse rolled me to I guess what you call, a surgery type room, and I'm told to slide over to a cold stainless table. Check your dignity at the door, there will be no secrets in here. I lie on a cold table, totally void of any clothes, and get informed they will now shave me of all hair anywhere near the entry area. At some point the doctor starts to work on my upper thigh. I can only assume that I'm given a mild sedative at some point because I never feel the catheter inserted into the artery in my leg. Through most of the procedure, I felt as though I am aware, seeing the monitor above me, seeing what I assumed was the catheter traveling through my body up to my heart. At no time was there ever any discomfort. My thoughts only went to re-assuring myself that all would be ok. At some point the doctor turned from his assistants to me. He advised me that I had a blocked artery. Just one that had a 99.1% blockage, and that I was very lucky to not have had a heart attack. "No crap doc! You've been telling me for four days there was nothing wrong." He informs me that he has inserted a stent in the blocked artery, and I should be as good as new.

> ***I will give you a new heart and put a new spirit in you; I will remove from you your heart of stone and give you a heart of flesh. (Ezekiel 36:26 NIV)***

It's funny how when we search out the words of God, he speaks. Each of the scriptures that I've chosen in this journal are scriptures not chosen by a bible scholar, but chosen by a normal everyday person such as yourself. As I write this journal, I try and give God my ear. Something I don't do enough. As I have done that, he has led me within his written word to scriptures that I feel fit within the pieces of my journey. I thank God that for his patience that even a 54 year old man that submits to him, can still hear his voice.

So here I am. Good as new. Rolling back to my room on a Thursday afternoon while having just experienced what could be deemed a life saving procedure. Feeling like a million bucks right? Sorry, but far from it. At this point, being appreciative of God's journey was not at the front of my mind. I think at this point, all of the emotions of the day came tumbling down on me. I wept uncontrollably. Couldn't tell you why at that point, but as I look back now, I think it was the realization of what I had just been through, and the reality of being near death. I had spent nearly a week acting and feeling like I was the epitome of health for a 54 year old guy. And suddenly, I realize like a flat on a tire, we've just put a patch on the ole ticker.

Now don't jump and criticize me here. I had just rolled out of a completely unplanned procedure that I never expected in a million years. Although my initial response may have seemed unappreciated, my appreciation for what you could describe as a second chance at life would come around very quickly. I had an artery, supplying life giving blood, OVER 99% blocked. God had to have a hand in allowing my heart to continue to operate without a heart attack.

The night following the angioplasty was a long one. The incision point, of where the catheter was inserted began to bleed uncontrollably because of the blood thinners they had me on. For the next 8 hours, a nurse sat by my bedside, holding pressure on the incision. Nothing like having someone poking a finger in an incision on your leg. Eventually, things got under control, and the cardio doctor finally got his wish of the week–to send me home.

He heals the broken hearted and binds up their wounds. (Psalm 147:3 NIV)

So this started my journey of 2013. On June 15th, God's hands directed a lifesaving stent into my body. Although I didn't experience the sudden burst of energy I've heard others describe, the pain I had experienced the last 6 months or so was gone. I became very appreciative of how lucky I was. I made a call to the Gastro doctor's office, and I passed word through the nurse that the PA's hunch had saved my life. So much for my "second team" comment. Life became "different". Cyndi and I became more aware of our life style. The rib eye steaks and fatty carb rich Cajun food became treats, instead of staples. The occasional beer, or drink, became virtually non-existent. Living at least semi-healthy became a lifestyle we had never truly embraced. Walking and biking became something we, at least for once, made an effort at.

Round 2

Left Brain

Now before we go any further I would like to explain something. As the title of this book describes, the meat of this story is about Stroke, not hearts and stents. Although the previous paragraphs dealt strictly with my heart and its blockage, I did that because I felt it was an integral part of my whole story of 2013. There will also be some similarities I'll explain that survivors and caregivers can be aware of, whether you are a stroke victim or recovering from some type of heart disease. Both afflictions leave a path of devastation that kills, disables, and breaks down the will to live of thousands per year.

Fast forward 5 months later to November 2013. I have had several follow-ups with my cardiologist at this point. Everything seems fine in his opinion. Although I'm dealing with the mental aspect of worrying about this foreign object stuck in my chest, I'm physically doing fine. I have occasional dull pains shoot through my chest, but I'm reassured by the doctor they are nothing other than my system reacting to an object in my artery. He tries to reassure me it's normal and will soon go away. Of course, I probably acerbate my worrying by doing my own research on the Internet. Google can be a wonderful and terrifying thing.

My health may fail, and my spirit grows weak, but God remains the strength of my Heart: he is mine forever. Psalms 73:26

November 16th–Cyndi is in New York with her niece Lori celebrating her daughter (Savannah's) 13th birthday. I get up at 7 am to go to a men's prayer breakfast at church. Weather is cloudy, but warm, so I decide to ride the Harley. One of my close friends, Ken Vaughn and I had discussed riding to Galveston for lunch, about a 45 minute ride. We meet at the church, have our get together, and eat wonderful bacon, eggs and other heart heathy grub. Now I will remind you of my journey so far this year. I have up to this point been doing a fairly good job of eating healthy and trying to take care of myself. This particular breakfast is a treat, not the norm. As we walk outside after breakfast, we notice a fine misty rain falling, and decide to call each other later and discuss our ride. I mount up and head home while the rain is starting to come down harder. The 5 minute ride is wet, but uneventful. I pull in the garage and grab a towel to dry the bike off. I go in the house, strip out of wet clothes, and put my robe on to watch some TV. This is where life changes. I'm sitting on the couch and out of nowhere (imagine the feeling when your foot goes to sleep) that prickly feeling, almost close to feeling like a vibration. Suddenly, without warning, this described feeling envelopes my right side, predominantly my foot, leg, arm/fingers and face. I'm kind of in a freakish shock at this point, not knowing what has occurred. My first thought is some type of pinched nerve. I get up and walk around. I go to the bathroom to look at myself in the mirror. Face is not drooping. Nah, not a stroke. I hop in and take a quick shower. My right hand is tingling more, it's weak. I realize stepping out of the shower, a loss in coordination. This isn't right. I get dressed and take two baby aspirin, just in case. Little did I understand at this point, that this could have killed me if I had experienced the wrong type of stroke. I call my RN sister Linda, who advises me to call 911. She doesn't have to ask me twice. 911 dispatches the call, and within 5 minutes a police officer is coming in the front door I've opened. The officer has me do several test, smiling, sticking tongue out, and squeezing his hands. All seem normal to him, and we wait for medics. They arrive in the next few minutes and repeat the same basic tests. Seems no one is convinced, at this moment that this is a stroke. Vitals taken, bp is 181 over 101. Wow, something wrong there. I've never had high blood pressure before. Without much coaxing, I agree to go to hospital. Initially they want to take me to Bayshore hospital, and I firmly decline. Take me to Methodist in the Houston Medical Center, (one of the top stroke centers in the U.S.) Off we go for my first ambulance ride ever. I, still to this day, remember the details of that ride. The scenery out the window on that rainy day. The thought of the drivers in the cars around me. Some wondering what my emergency was. The texting of several church friends and family, just so someone besides my sister who is 2 hours away, knows where I am. The starting of an IV and thinking to myself, is this all silly?

Will I be home in a few hours watching TV thinking how stupid all this is? I probably pinched a nerve, and it's going to disappear just as I get to the hospital. Denial is a funny thing.

In we roll to the Methodist ER. A flurry of nurses and doctors converge on me. Bp, heart rate, blood sugar, EKG, off to CAT scan. Squeeze my hands, smile, stick your tongue out, hold your arms up, walk, sit stand. Initial CAT scan results come back, and guess what? Are you ready? No sign of a stroke! See! What did I say! Will be back in my recliner before the afternoon is out. Not so fast mister. We want to observe you....so much for my recliner. About this time, my RN sister arrives in the ER. Squeeze my hands, smile, stick out your tongue, hold your arms out, sit stand. I feel like a poodle at the Westminster Dog show I'm getting so many commands barked at me. In walks the Neurosurgeon, who confirms that the CAT scan did not indicate a Stroke, but from all symptoms added up, he still suspects I may have had one. Because of the Plavix and baby aspirin I'm on, he says they will not be giving me the lifesaving stroke drug t-Pa.

The only FDA approved treatment for ischemic strokes is tissue plasminogen activator (tPA,

also known as IV rtPA, given through an IV in the arm). tPA works by dissolving the clot and improving flow to the part of the brain being deprived of flow. If administered within 4.5 hours in eligible patients, tPA may improve the chances of recovering from a stroke.
(www.strokeassociation.org)

The doctor feels the drugs I'm on are enough. He orders a MRI of the brain, which he says will give a more detailed picture of what is going on. At this point, they advise me I'm being admitted.

Now keep in mind, at this point Cyndi my wife is in New York, and has no idea any of this has gone on. I've intentionally not called her to alarm her until we know more. I finally make that call, and I tell her I'm in Methodist, what happened, and that the CAT scan came up negative for a stroke, but they are keeping me for observation. When we hang up, she immediately calls my sister who backs up my story.

Over the next 24 hours, I'm poked, prodded, and everything imaginable. Another CAT scan, MRI and things I've probably forgotten at this point. Mentally, the stroke has not seemed to have had any effect on me. Physically, I still have numbness in my hand, arm and face. I have no idea at this point, how lucky I've been. The next day, Sunday, becomes a waiting game waiting for the doctors to decide a plan of action. Cyndi has a flight in from New York, which is scheduled to arrive around 3:30. Linda, my sister spent the night to keep an eye on me. Around 2:00, Dr Abraham, the neurologist, shows up. MRI confirms I did have a stroke. I had what was called an Ischemic Stroke, which is the most common of strokes. A blood clot traveled to my brain, on the left side. I questioned the doctor on what caused it. And he gives a variety of possibilities, including the option of being connected with my stent surgery 5 months earlier. He says there's no actual way to pinpoint where the stroke comes from, although all test including a ultrasound of the heart don't indicate any other clots in my system. This is the beginning of my education on the mysteries of the brain and strokes. How, in this day and age, with the miracles of medicine, could we be so clueless on an event that happens day in and day out in hospitals? We can operate on babies, in their mothers' wombs, but can't explain an everyday occurrence such as a stroke?

> **But there is a spirit in man, and the breath of the Almighty giveth them understanding. (Job 32:8 ASV)**

Cyndi arrives at the hospital around 5:00 Sunday afternoon. Such a relief to see her after a very eventful weekend you might say. The news that I did indeed have a stroke was broken to me while she was in flight from New York to Houston. So the first news I have to break to her is yes, I did have a stroke. She spends the night with me that night, which is a wonderful relief to me. Monday, they send in occupational, speech and physical therapist to evaluate my deficits. All in all, I'm in pretty good shape. No riding the Harley for a while, but other than that the neurologist tells me to stay home the rest of the week and see him the following Monday. Deficits at this point are numbness and weakness on my right side. Numbness and tingling in my right cheek and mouth. One thing that I have a lot of trouble with is emotions which is quickly diagnosed as something termed PBA.

> **"Pseudo Bulbar Affect (PBA) is a medical condition characterized by sudden and**

uncontrollable episodes of crying or laughing. It is sometimes referred to as emotional lability, pathological crying and laughing or emotional incontinence. An episode of PBA can occur at any time, even in inappropriate social situations.

PBA can occur in stroke survivors or people with other neurologic conditions such as dementia, multiple sclerosis, Lou Gehrig's disease (ALS) or traumatic brain injury. It is thought to affect more than 1 million people in the U.S. PBA is often mistaken for depression, causing it to be under-diagnosed, under-treated and sometimes inappropriately treated." (www.support.stroke.org)

I will tell you now, as a survivor of stroke, this was one of the hardest things I had to deal with, especially being a man. Although there was a confirmed reason for these emotional outburst (mine were all crying), dealing with this was extremely hard. I could hardly carry on a conversation at church with friends without wanting to burst into tears. This was a huge embarrassment for me. The good news was, as soon as we discussed this with the neurologist, medication was prescribed that pretty much cured the problem. One thing we learned about what we were going through, and I say we because obviously my loved ones travelled this path with me, was that no question was sacred with my doctors. Asking the simplest, hardest, most embarrassing questions was the only way to get answers.

So home I go on Monday. **Official diagnoses – Acute 1cm infarction of the left thalamus.** No therapy prescribed. No real restrictions. Only medicine change is blood pressure meds. Reality begins to set in. The first week at home, my mind tends to be on overtime. The reality of having a stroke really sets in. The why and the worry of what if it happens again start to consume me. My MD and neurologist both try to assure this won't happen again. Although they are very convincing, I can't seem to put it to rest that I'm really ok. I'm given anti-depressants to try and relieve my worries. These help some, but are not a cure all. Fear comes in many forms. Mine is a fear of history repeating itself.

Sleepless nights. The brain is an amazing machine. Dreams seem so real. Dreams of good and bad.

I saw a dream which made me afraid; and the thoughts upon my bed and the visions of my head troubled me. (Daniel 4:5 ASV)

Today as I sit here writing, I sit beside my mom in the nursing home who is slowly slipping away under hospice care. It's funny, because just a little over a year ago I sat beside Cyndi's mom Eloise in the same situation. Here is an elderly person, who's lived a long life, laying here in this bed just waiting for the Lord to take her hand. In between the doses of morphine is very little coherent conversation. Living in a drug induced dreamland. What goes through your mind at this point? Here you are, standing at the edge of this world. Family all comes to say their last goodbyes, even though they don't say that. Sleep. Fog. You just exist on the edge of earth. Heaven is just a breath away, you just don't know which breath. I guess when thinking about it, that's no different than our whole life. We all stand one breath away from that eternal end. We just don't except that as being real. We live as though there is a tomorrow. Even though that's never been guaranteed.

Boast not thyself of tomorrow; for thou knowest not what a day may bring forth. (Proverbs 27:1 ASV)

So Monday, I'm discharged. I must say, Cyndi wasn't near as happy as I. We are going home with no real answers of "why". All we know is, I had a stroke. An Ischemic Stroke, the most common. Was it connected to my stent back in June? Or, did it just happen to be from plaque in an Artery that just happened to break loose. Thus we begin, the unknown of a typical stroke patient.

It's been 11 days since I wrote in this journal. Although this journal was started to document my experiences over the last year of heart and stroke issues, I pause here. I pause to write about a sweet mother, who 11 days ago, holding mine and my sister's hand gasped her last breath before our very eyes. I saw at that moment the miracle of death. A body, a machine created by a God some say, created by celestial colliding of neutrons, say others. Either, from the surface, seemingly unbelievable events. Only by Faith do those of us who believe in God, do we understand that the unbelievable is completely believable. A God that has always been and that will always be. I would say some have been amazed, at how few emotions I exhibited during this event. Some worry that I'm holding things in. Sometimes I worry too. But from what I feel, I think that I'm truly at peace with my earthly mother returning to the heavenly father above. A wonderful journey just shy of 89 years. From the little girl that wandered hand in hand with her best friend Margie into Eastwood Baptist church, and obediently answered an alter call to baptism. To an old woman, who fulfilled a complete life. Using every bit of energy that God blessed that body with, down to that last breath. She hurts no more. She worries no more. She has everything she could ever want and need now. She's with her earthly momma again, her earthly father, her brothers and her sisters. Her and her birth family, together again. I'll miss mom, but I feel comfort in knowing where she is.

The Lord is my shepherd; I shall not want. He maketh me to lie down in green pastures: he leadeth me beside the still waters. He restoreth my soul: he leadeth me in the paths of righteousness for his name's sake. Yea, though I walk through the valley of the shadow of death, I will fear no evil: for thou art with me; thy rod and thy staff they comfort me. Thou preparest a table before me in the presence of mine enemies: thou anointest my head with oil; my cup runneth over. Surely goodness and mercy shall follow me all the days of my life: and I will dwell in the house of the Lord for ever. (Psalms 23:1-6 KJV)

So the unknown happened. I know I had a stroke, but don't know why. I don't know if it's because of my stent, which I take Plavix for. I don't know if it's because of my high blood pressure, which I take Amlodipine, and Lisinopril for. I don't know if it's because of my cholesterol, which I take Pravistatin for and I don't know if it's because of some other reason the doctor hasn't pin pointed. So I take 9 pills in the morning, and 3 pills at night, and I lie awake getting anxiety attacks wondering if that little pain I just felt is the next big one. Silly you say? I assure you from the eyes of a stroke survivor not. Fear. Fear of death. Fear of permanent incapacitation. Yes I know, there are thousands of other afflictions to the human that can inject this fear. But we're dealing with me. Not ready to retire. At least 10 more years to work. Baseballs to throw my grand kids. So who has time for a stroke? A catastrophic attack to the body. Slurred speech, droopy face. Limbs that don't operate. Unable to walk normally, much less run as I was doing days before.

So we very quietly, arrive home from Methodist hospital to await what's next. I do know, at this point I'm very lucky. Lucky to be alive. Lucky to have as few a deficits as I do from the stroke. Weakness on my right side. Tingling/ numbness in my right hand and face. I had the preverbal close call. I'm thankful. I'm at this point appreciating the fact that things could have been much worse. It's Tuesday, November 19th, 2013. Dr. Thomas instructs me to at least take off until Friday. The following week is only a three-day week due to Thanksgiving. Black Friday, Cyndi and I are scheduled to fly to Arkansas to visit her niece in Russellville, Arkansas. I put light effort into working the three days before thanksgiving, have our family get together and gorge on Turkey and everything else associated with the day. Family is a special treat for me this Thanksgiving. Lots to have thanks for.

> ***I will praise the name of God with a song, and will magnify him with thanksgiving. (Psalms 69:30 KJV)***

Round 3
Right Brain

Black Friday, 2013. Cyndi and I drive to Hobby Airport to catch our Southwest flight to Littlerock, to where we will rent a car and drive the 2 hours to Russellville. Looking back, maybe God gave us a small sign before we even got started. We get to the airport, and there is not a parking spot to be found in any lot, nor even any hotel around the airport. We drive around for an hour. Nothing. Finally, her niece Lori comes to the rescue, leaving my truck at a Denny's, and Lori dropping us at the airport. A close call, but all is well, and we make our flight. An uneventful flight to Littlerock, an uneventful drive to Russellville. We settle in for what we intend to be, a relaxing weekend overlooking the Arkansas River at the home of Deanna, her niece.

We are a hardheaded species aren't we? We go on, day by day, as if we will live forever. Then, that one crisis invades our life, and we become full of insight, critical of ourselves and our selfishness of time. But then, as most crisis pass, we become complacent with life again. Slipping back into our selfish lives. Do we learn? Of course, God blessed us with that ability. But like freshman algebra, the big picture starts to fade. Only that which is required is retained. I'll never need that.

The furthest thing on my mind at this point is having another issue. I'm done, with nothing to do but recover. We go sight seeing up to the top of Mount Nebo. We sit on the back porch watching mount Nebo in the distance. Beautiful sunsets from the back deck. The Arkansas River far below the cliffs behind the house. College football bowl games, one after another. Rest and relaxation is just what is needed. Monday rolls around and our niece Deanna takes her husband Dave to the doctor to have a knee X-ray, due to a motorcycle accident he had the day we arrived. Cyndi and I leisurely get up, pack and eat breakfast. Our flight is at 7:00 that evening, which will be preceded by dinner with our friends

Scott and Farah Gray who just moved to Littlerock. Cyndi has her shower, and settles in to watch TV while I get ready. Peaceful, quiet morning. I jump in for a hot shower.

> **Moreover, no one knows when their hour will come: As fish are caught in a cruel net, or birds are taken in a snare, so people are trapped by evil times that fall unexpectedly upon them. (Ecclesiastes 9:12 NIV)**

Blood thinners, Plavix, baby aspirin, blood pressure meds, etc. We have everything covered Dr. Thomas said. "YOU DO NOT NEED TO WORRY ABOUT ANOTHER STROKE" he says. As I stand in the shower, a feeling hits me. Not exactly as before. But a feeling of dread. A feeling of, something's wrong. A thickness invades my tongue. My left leg and arm become heavy. This can't be. I'm imagining this. It will pass, the water was maybe just too hot. I get out of the shower and dry. My lips are numb. Come on Louis, your minds playing with you. I dress. Walk past Cyndi who's watching TV. No need to panic her. This is nothing. I'll walk it off. I go out the front door, to walk down the driveway, and up the hill a ways.

As I come back down the hill, my coordination is definitely off. My left leg is not working, as it should. Looking back, the going outside part was really pretty stupid. I come back into the house, and I'm not really sure what I did next. But, I ended up telling Cyndi "something's wrong". She stares at me in disbelief. What do you mean? I mean my tongue is thick, I'm having trouble talking and walking. Cyndi says, "Do you need to go to the hospital?" I don't remember if I said yes, the first time she asked, but eventually I did. Are you serious? She says. "Louis we're in Russellville, Arkansas. You want to go to the hospital here?" Now all of you who read this must understand, we had nothing against Arkansas hospitals, we are just used to the Texas Medical Center, the facility's that treat people from all over the world. I don't think this hospital in Russellville, Arkansas has a lot of international travelers flocking to it. Well, we need to do something I say. A quick call to our niece, and they decided it would be best just to put me in the car and drive me down the mountain to the hospital. Cyndi loads the car with our bags, then me, and we start to drive. I don't remember a lot of details of that drive, other than fear setting in. I remember my emotions taking over my thoughts. And thinking here we go again. Only difference this time is I know something serious is happening. I pretty much knew, during that drive down, that I had another stroke. Cyndi pulls up to the emergency entrance of St Mary's hospital, and I get out so she can park the car. I walked in on my own, walking to the receptionist who asks, "can I help you?" I respond "I'm having a stroke". To which the receptionist responds kind of in a unbelieving tone "how do you know?" To which I respond, "I just had one three weeks ago." She seemed to believe me at that point and a nurse comes around and leads me to triage.

Have mercy on me, Lord, for I am faint; heal me, Lord, for my bones are in agony. (Psalm 6:2 NIV)

Here we go again–blood pressure, IV, stick your tongue out, lift your leg, squeeze my finger, on, and on. I'm immediately put on a stretcher and wheeled to a CAT scan. One thing I'll say for them, they wasted no time. I'm rolled back into the ER treatment room to await results. Emotions really kick in now, and I have to tell you, I sobbed. This can't be happening again. This is not real. What is this now God? What are you trying to teach me? Cyndi does her best to calm me. The doctor comes in and gets Cyndi and takes her to look at a computer screen. Obviously, showing her the CAT scan of this stroke. They and the conversation, wander my way. They've confirmed I've had another Stroke. Not the same type of stroke, but a Hemorrhagic stroke, similar to an aneurism. A bleeder, they call it. On top of this, it's on the opposite side of the brain from the first Stroke. No t-Pa again, the life saving drug that saves the lives of so many stroke victims. My problem now basically, is my blood is too thin from the Plavix and aspirin. I'm given a shot of vitamin K which helps thicken the blood. Cyndi tells the doctor, "No offense but I want him transferred to a bigger hospital that can treat this." The Doctor gives no argument, "There's really not much we can do for him here". I'm informed they are calling Life Flight from St Vincent's hospital in Littlerock, to transfer me. Which is about a 90-mile trip by ground. An hour and a half drive. The air transfer will take 30 minutes for the copter to arrive and another 30-45 minutes back. Cyndi and her niece Deanna will have to make the trip by car.

I said, "Oh, that I had the wings of a dove! I would fly away and be at rest. (Psalm 55:6 NIV)

I would imagine, we all have wondered, what it would be like to fly in a Life flight helicopter. I know I have. Although, what has to happen to get that ride we would never wish on anyone including ourselves. It was kind of funny, everyone involved wore a helmet, except me. I guess they figure my brain is scrambled enough at this point. I meet the pilots and the nurse who will be monitoring me. I want to sit up front by the pilot, but he declines. I'm wheeled outside the hospital, and loaded up. Through everything I've been through, this is no big deal to me. Flying is actually something I love. Although I'm very calm, this ride gives me time to reflect on what's happening. As we lift off, I see Cyndi and Deanna video taping the helicopter takeoff. I close my eyes, and pray to God, that he protects Cyndi and the boys. I know there is fear among us all of how this day will end. As I fly towards Little Rock, I view the beautiful countryside. I'm thinking its beauty is nothing to what we will see in heaven. I think of my grandbabies, and how I look forward to them sitting in my lap, hugging my neck. I'm peacefully calm through the 45-minute ride. I have no idea what's in store next. Therapy, surgery, drugs, test after test. How will we get home? The ride comes to a gentle end. The next phase of my journey is about to start.

May your unfailing love be with us, Lord, even as we put our hope in you. (Psalm 33:22 NIV)

Funny, the landing of the helicopter and what came next was nothing as I pictured. I had it worked out to look like the TV show MASH. Doctors and nurses standing on the Tarmac, and wash from the helicopter blowing everything in sight. Nurses trying to hold their hats on and dresses down. Everyone ducking running under the blades to get to the trauma patient. Reality, the helicopter gently sits down on the pad. I hear the engines shut down, and the blades come to a slow stop. Two nurses come to meet the helicopter crew, and calmly wheel me into the emergency room. Welcome to Little Rock Arkansas, specifically, St. Vincent Infirmary Hospital, and your home for the near future.

My destination is the Neuro ICU. I'm wheeled in, and the usual test start. You know–Bp, heart rate, squeeze this, what's your name, what day is it. Probably the highlight was the insertion of an arterial Blood Pressure device, which is basically an IV. Inserted into an artery in the arm that gives a constant Blood Pressure read out. I would have to say, the male nurse that took the first three "stabs" at inserting this caused me the most pain of the last year. Finally, a female anesthesiologist comes in, and gets it first try. Cyndi and Deanna arrive about this time from their drive from Russellville. Emotions for me are running high, and it was good to see familiar faces. I'm wheeled to X-ray for another CAT scan, to make sure the vessel in my brain has not continued to leak. Although, I'm totally aware, and coherent, I have definite paralysis on my left side. The ability to take my left index finger and touch my nose does not exist. Paralysis from the first stroke still provides major numbness to my right side, including my hand, face, lips and inner mouth. I require assistance eating, drinking, peeing, and well, you know. Current CAT scan indicates no further leakage. **Official diagnoses – Right Cerebral Hemorrhage. Hemorrhage measures at least 3.1 cm in transverse diameter, and up to 3.5 cm in craniocaudad length, and 2 cm in diameter.** We'll repeat the cat-scan at 4 am everyday for the next week. I'll be glowing for the next year from all of the radiation.

For the next few days, attention is aimed at controlling blood pressure. Meds are adjusted pretty continually while trying to get me down to a manageable range. Novalox shots are given in my stomach twice a day, to help manage the thickness of my blood.

Although, I spend almost a week in ICU, most of what I remember was non-eventful. Everything became pretty routine. Eat, TV, eat, bath, TV, eat, and snack. This is when boredom really set in. I'll have to say, if it wasn't for some of the nurses having a personality, and their ability to joke back and forth with me, I would have gone nuts. Mid-week, I have Cyndi get an edible arraignment for the nurses, which scores big in getting attention. Also, about mid-week, Cyndi helps one of the nurses discover my Afrin nose spray, which I've sort of been hiding. I get a good lecture from the nurse, who suggests I make the Afrin disappear. Afrin was something I had been hooked on for probably 30 years. I took my last sniff in that hospital room and haven't reached for it since. Later, it's explained to me that Afrin can cause thinning of the mucous membranes in the nose, and could possibly, although not likely, play a factor in a stroke. That's what they told me anyways.

Mid- week, we started getting out of bed and walking with a walker. Me, I thought I was ready to run. My body put me in check. Picking my feet up became the phrase of the week. My left leg tended to drag if I didn't think about it. I progressed well, even though I wouldn't be running anytime soon.

Four days into my ICU stay, they move me to a regular room. That Thursday afternoon, I had the most wonderful shower of my life. Cyndi had to assist, but just to get my hair washed was exhilarating. Cyndi's brother Pat arrives to assist us in getting home. By this time of course, Cyndi had cancelled our flights home and even turned our rent car in. I must mention also, this was during the time of one of the worst winters the mid-west had seen. More freezing rain and record cold were predicted for the next couple of days. Pat and I went into overtime trying to convince the doctors, it was time to send me home. Cyndi was not in any hurry to check me out. Obviously, she was considering the long road ahead.

Friday, with the assurance I would get therapy in Houston and get directly to a neurologist for direction, we were told I could check out and head home. We were instructed that it would not be advisable to fly, but that had already been taken care of with Pats arrival. So, bags packed and we head to the hotel next door for my last night in Little Rock Arkansas.

If you do this and God so commands, you will be able to stand the strain, and all these people will go home satisfied." (Exodus 18:23 NIV)

Saturday morning, chance of ice, snow and rain. We wake to temps in the low 20's, but radio reports of the ice and snow being minimal. Cyndi, is a nervous wreck, but all turns out for the best. Freeways are fairly clear with the threat of what could have been passing to the north of Little Rock and sparing us. We tread on starting our 8 hour journey towards home. Arriving home around 4:00 in the afternoon, I'm greeted by our two shitzus and my recliner. This will be my docking station, for the next 3-4 weeks, as we go into recovery mode.

So where do we stand at this point? From the first stroke, I still have numbness in my right hand, fingers, in my face and lips. I have a high sensitivity to my skin. Even using a q-tip to clean my ears sends sharp pains through my body. Now, added from the second stroke, I have a profound weakness to my left side. My leg and arm are noticeably weak. Coordination and use of my left hand are definitely impaired. Holding things in my hand are near impossible. Dropping things becomes a daily and

Right Brain

highly frustrating act. Cyndi hears words come from my mouth that she shouldn't hear, when my frustration takes over. Speech is strained. My volume, at which I speak, is a near whisper. Taste buds are off, due to my tongue being numb. To say the least, I'm a jumbled up mess. Don't get me wrong though, I realize how lucky I am. I realize how bad this could have been. I could be paralyzed. I could be on a ventilator. I could be deaf or blind. I could be.......... dead. But God has further plans for me.

Monday starts recovery. Monday resting is over. Time to get to work.

> ***May the favor of the Lord our God rest on us; establish the work of our hands for us— yes, establish the work of our hands. (Psalm 90:17 NIV)***

Round 4

Recovery

December 9, 2013–Stroke recovery begins. Cyndi is given the rest of the month off from her job she's only been at 3 months. Another blessing. A truly Godly run company. USD corp was truly a blessing in our lives at this point. She's able to concentrate on what I/we need to do. Monday morning the phone calls begin. Appointments with neurologist, cardiologist, MD and look for therapist. As far as we know, I'll need occupational, physical, and speech therapy. Our first appointment of the week is with Dr Abraham, my neurologist. Dr.Abraham is the doctor who told me to quit worrying about another stroke. All the meds I'm on have everything in check. Boy is he surprised by my story on this visit. Dr. Abraham exhibits true empathy. He understands. He makes you feel as though he is truly sorry for what you're going through. A trait, I would like to master.

> **em·pa·thy noun \\'em-pə-thē**
> **: the feeling that you understand and share another person's experiences and emotions : the ability to share someone else's feelings**
> "www.merrian-webster.com"

In the next months, I will experience much sympathy instead of empathy. The difference? I guess the best way to describe it is people who exhibit empathy towards a situation, try to just understand, not understand and try to explain how lucky you are. Just because you think I "look" great, doesn't mean I am. And just because you "say" I look great, doesn't mean I believe you. In other words, I don't need you to help me feel better. I just need you to understand how I feel. I need you to try to understand what I've been through, even though you may not be capable. I really need you to understand that what you see, may not be what I feel. I, even today, want to scream, when people say how great I look. I want to yell, "I feel like crap, I can't feel my fingers, lips and tongue. So it doesn't matter, how I <u>look</u> to you." Don't assume. I know. People mean well. They truly do. I just ask that you think before you speak, before you try to lift up a person. Sometimes, all people need to hear is that you understand and are truly sorry for what they've gone through. Not point out the bright side to them.

New symptom of my stroke–high sensitivity, sensitive nerve endings, face hurts to touch and gums hurt to brush. It's as though my nerve endings in certain parts of my body have their volume turned up to high. Lyrica prescribed.

So just for your info. Maybe I should summarize all of my deficits as I start this recovery. Remember now, some of these are from the first stroke and some from the second. At this point, I'll just summarize them all together.

1. Weakness in left leg, arm and hand–this has me using a cane/walker at this point. Attempts to walk without result in leg dragging, causing fall threat. Arm weakness causes severe incoordination in doing things such as using TV remote, combing hair and buttoning shirts. Hand deficits cause inability to grasp

and hold items. Attempts to do so result in many dropped items. Much frustration because of this.

2. Weakness/ numbness in right hand. More hand/eye coordination problems with things such as remote, grasping and holding. Numbness causes an inability to feel things, such as picking up a penny off a table. Imagine, if you can, your worse case of foot or hand falling asleep. That tingly pins and needles feeling. That describes the feeling, except it doesn't go away.

3. Numbness in lips/tongue/gums. Results in reduced inability to taste. This will be one of my most disappointing deficits, but maybe at the same time one of my largest blessings. I'll explain this later.

4. Dryness to facial skin and eyes. Very annoying due to being contact wearer for most my life. Left eye especially dries out.

5. Pain in fingers of right hand. Maybe described as similar to arthritis. Although I've never been diagnosed with arthritis before, so I'm only guessing. I can only describe as a bone deep pain in my fingers. Probably the most painful of all deficits. One that eventually partially drives me to sell my beloved Harley Davidson.

6. Impaired speech. Vocals at a level barely above a whisper. This is a deficit I cannot acknowledge without my speech therapist. To me, I was talking normal. Speech is sometimes slurred.

7. Some memory issues. Although, most are more memory skills and ability to solve.

> *I cried like a swift or thrush, I moaned like a mourning dove. My eyes grew weak as I looked to the heavens. I am being threatened; Lord, come to my aid!" (Isaiah 38:14 NIV)*

So for the most part, these are my problems. Obviously, defining my goals to overcome. Some, I will overcome easily. Some possibly, never. A scary thought.

My regiment of prescriptions at this point = 8 pills, including.

1. Lisinoprole–blood pressure
2. Plavix – Stent Maintenance
3. Nuedexta–Emotions
4. Wellbutrin–Depression
5. Gabapentin – Nerve endings

6. Atorvastin–Cholesterol

7. Pantoprazole – Acid reflux

8. CoQ10 – Muscle aches

I said I would explain this later, but tonight I feel compelled to write about this. Tonight I treated myself to what used to be one of my favorite meals, a bacon sandwich. Although, normally a homemade meal, this particular one was ordered from Subway. With no fault to Subway, it was horrible. As I said before, one of my most disappointing deficits is my ability to taste. I always felt I had a pretty good pallet for food, and that for now has been totally devastated by these strokes. Favorite meals, such as steak, sushi and the flavorful Cajun foods I've learned to love, now for the most part do very little for me pleasure wise. Foods are now just memories, and eating just sustains life. Tonight, it really hit me while eating that sandwich, how much I used to enjoy the taste of foods. Now it dawns on me, that pleasure, was an empty addiction. Something that gave instant pleasure, but had very little substance to life. Those pleasures, especially the most decadent ones, were the most damaging substances that entered my mouth, creating much of the position I'm in. High blood pressure, high cholesterol, etc. Although there were other circumstances that led to my turn in health, food was the number one cause.

So, we have to find the silver lining in all our circumstances right? Mine has to be to learn, that food, cannot and will not be used as pleasure, but as a necessity for life. God actually blessed me with this particular deficit. Before my heart stent, almost exactly one year ago, I weighed 207lbs. The heaviest I had ever been in my life. Today, I step on the scale at 167lbs, and weight continues to come off slowly. Although most foods, no longer give me the pleasures I once had, I enjoy having the control over eating I once lacked. I'm living healthier, and have more energy. A silver lining. God is good.

> ***I will give you hidden treasures, riches stored in secret places, so that you may know that I am the Lord, the God of Israel, who summons you by name. (Isaiah 45:3 NIV)***

Work begins. One week after returning home from Arkansas, therapy starts. The physical part I was prepared for. Strength, coordination, all had to be honed. These were easy for me. Although

I was never a super athlete, competition was in my blood. I've always loved a good challenge. Squats, leg presses, curls, and anything else they could think of, I breezed through. Coordination exercises, proved a little more challenging, but nothing I couldn't handle. The real test came when speech therapy started. This is where Priya stepped in, my speech therapist. The most important rehabilitation of my life, would be lead by her. Exercising mentally was more taxing than any mile run they could send me on. I knew how to push my body physically. But pushing my brain, was much harder. First test–draw the face of a clock, with the time 3:00 on it. Couldn't do it. Couldn't fit the 12 numbers where they go. That's when I realized, how damaged I really was. Emotions were high.

Problem solving was really difficult too. Her simple test revealed to me the complexity of my affliction. Her assurance to me that mental exercise, would improve all, gave me hope. Priyas diagnoses Dysarthria, which is a motor speech disorder resulting from neurological injury of the motor component of the motor-speech system and is characterized by poor articulation.

Priya puts me to work, drilling me with exercises to stimulate my brain, giving me homework. She also gives me physical exercise for the tongue, cheeks and mouth, to try and stimulate the nerve endings. Part of my brain has died, but with the right stimulation, the brain is a marvelous machine that will rewrite itself. My prognosis at this point, is hopeful, although there are no guarantees with brain injuries. Recovery at this point, is really not more than 50/50. Priya assures me, we will work hard to overcome though. Priya has a unique way of making you believe. I walk away from my first session hopeful.

Guide me in your truth and teach me, for you are God my Saviour, and my hope is in you all day long. (Psalm 25:5 NIV)

So in the following weeks, life revolves around therapy. Three hours a day, three days a week. I'm training for a Marathon, a run for the rest of my life. All of it is grueling. I challenge all of my therapist to challenge me. I want to get through this, and be normal again, whatever that is. Although the physical therapy is challenging at times, I really enjoy the accomplishments that quickly come from my work. Occupational therapy is another story, boring, frustrating. My hands and their numbness will be the hardest to overcome. Coordination comes slow. My expectation of this therapy comes the lowest. Speech, is totally different. Hard for me to measure. Accomplishments much harder for me to see. Priya and Cyndi are my cheer leaders, and the encouragement they give, the praise that they give, are the only thing keeping me going. Having encouragement is immeasurable at this time. Progress in all areas is measured in baby steps. I eventually shed my cane, which was the crutch of balance. Graduate to a stair stepper, treadmill and eventually the stairwell in the building. It's amazing what a little hard work can accomplish. In occupational therapy, we come to an impasse. My biggest problem, is feeling in my fingers. I think we came to the realization that this would just take time. I accomplish all goals, but some things as I said, will just have to work themselves out in time. A few days before New Years, 2013, I'm discharged from occupational and physical therapy. I have one more appointment for 2013 schedule with Priya, who was on vacation my last two appointments. My expectation is she's going to want to continue therapy 4-6 sessions starting the New Year. January 31st, New Year's Eve, Priya gives me the ultimate encouragement, on the last day of one of the most challenging years of my life, she tells me we are done. I cry like a baby. We hug, and I tell her what an Angel she is. God truly blessed this young woman with a talent. She sends me out, ready to start living again. New Years Day 2014, a time for true new beginnings.

> ***Jesus replied, "Very truly I tell you, no one can see the kingdom of God unless they are born again. " (John 3:3 NIV)***

How fitting this verse is for me at this time in my life. Although, I'm already a born again believer, the term "born again" has brought a whole new meaning that I have yet to understand. As I write this, I'm coming up on the 1 year anniversary of my heart stent. The 6 month anniversary of my second stroke. Even today, I continue to understand the words that Priya told me. "You are not the same person you were, you will have to find the new you." She also told me that I will have ups, and downs, maybe 6 months or longer. Such a wise young woman. Boy, have there been ups and downs. The problem with the downs are, I struggle alone with them. I can't explain them to anyone. My mind plays these games of tricking me to think that next stroke is around the corner. I have good days and bad. Numbness, weakness, inability to articulate and inability to taste. The bad days take a toll. They cause bad moods, depression and physical exhaustion. I take it out on the ones I love. I struggle, to pull myself up, and press on. My job some times is the only saving of my sanity. As a Salesman, I'm forced to flip that switch in front of a customer. That switch that turns on the charm, that everything is all right. I'm here to be your happy savior of your problems, what can I do for you? But you can only run on that adrenalin for so long. Eventually you come back to reality–I've had a stroke. I've been reborn. I'm a new person, whether I like it or not. Whatever was normal for me, is no longer. I am the NEW normal, whatever that is.

He put a new song in my mouth, a hymn of praise to our God. Many will see and fear the Lord and put their trust in him. (Psalm 40:3 NIV

So I'm one year into this journey. To recap, during this year I've had a near heart attack that resulted in a stent. An Ischemic Stroke, while my wife was away in New York. A Hemorrhagic stroke while on vacation in Arkansas. I dealt with my wife having a blood clot go to her kidney, and most recently, dealt with the loss of my 89-year-old mom. Quite a year I would have to say. Life goes on though. Even though life has changed for me, I accept that I still have a job to do on this place we call earth. Until my heavenly father calls me home, I'll continue to adapt and persevere at whatever is thrown my way. My taste buds are my biggest challenge, but with that comes a loss of 40 lbs., that makes me feel and look healthier. My right hand is numb, but function-able. Very slight weakness in both hands still exists. Opening or tearing things sometimes require assistance. Left leg is still slightly weak, with minor coordination issues, but I can run on a treadmill, and exercise on an elliptical. I still have bouts of fear that set in quit often, of subsequent strokes. And let's don't forget hidden heart issues that started this journey. Every little headache makes me worry. Depression bouts still exist, although I feel like I'm learning to cope better every day. I take my 8 pills a day religiously. Most of all, I talk to God daily. If anyone understands, I know he does. I could not have survived this without my faith. Faith in doctors. Faith in Cyndi. Faith in modern medicine. Most of all, faith in my Lord and Savior.

Statistics

Stroke kills almost 130,000 Americans each year—that's 1 out of every 19 deaths.

On average, one American dies from stroke every 4 minutes.

Every year, more than 795,000 people in the United States have a stroke.

About 610,000 of these are first or new strokes.

About 185,00 strokes—nearly one of four—are in people who have had a previous stroke.

About 87% of all strokes are ischemic strokes, when blood flow to the brain is blocked.

"www.cdc.gov"

Americans suffer 1.5 million heart attacks and strokes each year. Cardiovascular disease—including heart disease and stroke—is the leading cause of death in the United States. Every day, 2,200 people die from cardiovascular diseases—that's nearly 800,000 Americans each year, or 1 in every 3 deaths.

"www.millionhearts.hhs.gov"

Worldwide Statistics

According to the World Health Organization, 15 million people suffer stroke worldwide each year. Of these, 5 million die and another 5 million are permanently disabled.

High blood pressure contributes to more than 12.7 million strokes worldwide.

Europe averages approximately 650,000 stroke deaths each year.

In developed countries, the incidence of stroke is declining, largely due to efforts to lower blood pressure and reduce smoking. However, the overall rate of stroke remains high due to the aging of the population.

"www.strokecenter.org"

July 27, 2014

It's Sunday night, and I lie in bed typing this. What a weekend. Twinges of headache. Low blood pressure, 105/60. Low heart rate, 50-55 avg. Saturday, Cyndi gets a call from a close co-worker. Her parents were involved in a head on car accident in Galveston with a drunk driver. The father was killed instantly. Then tonight, Cyndi gets a text from her cousin from Louisiana who was just here for a visit. Seems a good friend, whom she visited while here in Houston, who was recovering from a stroke, died in her sleep. Why does death shock us so? I mean, it's one of the few things in life that we are guaranteed. It's going to happen, to every one of us. And those of us who profess to be Christian, or even just religious, believing in a higher power, shouldn't we rejoice at death? Because if we really truly believe, what we say we believe, we are all going to a much better place. That father, who died in that car wreck, he's walking the golden streets of heaven, without a worry, ever again. That young lady, who struggled from stroke deficits, is perfect again. Easy to say, much tougher to give our thoughts to, 100%.

> **For God so loved the world that he gave his one and only Son, that whoever believes in him shall not perish but have eternal life. (John 3:16 NIV)**

December 14, 2014

5 Months since writing in the journal that started this. Life moves on and consumes us. Life re-defines itself. Although my deficits haven't changed much in the last 5 months, the focuses on those deficits have somewhat blurred. The one year anniversary of each of my strokes have just past. Not much has changed physically or mentally which was related to the strokes. Thoughts still wander at times to the issues I live with. Depression and anxiety maybe aren't as prevalent. At times, I'm short tempered, which may or may not be stroke related. Dental work triggered a new issue to deal with. An injection in my lower left jaw for a crown, triggered Neuralgia. Definition – Neuralgia describes a variety of rare and painful conditions in which shooting, stabbing, pain occurs along the course of a nerve, usually in the head or neck. During the last 2-3 months we have attempted to treat the pain with several oral medications. During the last month, I've seen an acupuncturist getting a dozen or so treatments. None of the above have had any effect on relieving the neck pain. Now I've gone full circle back to my Neurologist, who is referring me

to a Pain Management specialist. If its not one thing, it's something else.

During the last 5 months, I've also found several outlets for my mental health. Although there are several stroke groups in my area I've attended, a handful of online stroke support groups on Facebook have been the most help. I highly suggest if you have access, get involved. Facebook groups such as – **(Second chance stroke survivors),(Life changes after stroke),** and my favorite, **(The stroke coffee house)** are truly therapeutic. Get involved. Don't just read, write. Talk about your stroke with people who have experienced what you have. You'll truly find people who understand. These are all people who have gone through what we have.

What now?

To my fellow stroke survivors

We move on my friends. We take each day, as we take each step. Sure footed, and deliberate. We realize, and accept right now, that some days will not be good, but we vow to cherish, the days that are. We educate, with compassion, our loved ones who try so hard to understand. Who act like they understand? Who have no idea that they don't understand at all. We try to understand ourselves that they, have been through a traumatic event too. They, have watched us struggle. Watched us cry. Watched us have bad days, and good. We are not alone in our pain. They hurt too. We have faith. Faith is complete trust or confidence, in someone, or something. Have faith in God. Faith in your doctors. Faith in yourself. We except who we are, and that we may not be, who we were. What is normal? Normal is what we are, even though normal may not be what it once was. Finally, but certainly far from the least, is how our strokes relate with those around us. Our spouses and those closest, deal with our deficits and us every day. As they try and relate, have patience, as we ask patience from them. Include them in your feelings. Include them in doctors' visits. Only being involved will they begin to understand our thoughts, our fears, and our wants. Those of us that are married, understand that marriage is hard enough sometimes. We have enough trouble understanding the opposite sex sometimes. But throw in a brain malady, that changes us overnight, and understanding is required at a new level. Be honest with your doctor with the struggles in this area. We need help from all, but can only get that help when we ask. My last advice – Journal. Find a way to put your feelings and thoughts down. This Journal/Book became the most incredible healing tool I could use.

To the Families of Stroke Survivors

This is hard. Really hard. Not only for them, but for you. You have been through a lot. What you have been through is not so different than what they have. You've been scared. You've been afraid. You fear losing your loved one. You fear subsequent events. You look into the eyes of your loved one, and don't know what to say. So ok, I've just listed everything you already know. What now? Talk. Tell them how you feel, and help them see that this is catastrophic for you too. Understand. Understand that this is the scariest thing they have ever gone through. Love. This is what you and they need most. Hug. Talk. Tell each other, that you're both going to be ok. Pray. Pray for each other. Pray for yourself. Pray that God gives you each peace. Calm. Patience. This will not be over quickly. Healing takes time. Days. Months. Yes, maybe even years. There will be good days. There will be some not so good.

Learn to take a deep breath during the rough times. Close your eyes, and ask God for calm, patience. You are not alone my friends. He who heals is watching. Blessing you. Giving you strength.

One thing my pastor James Johnson taught me through this was to grasp bible verses that speak to you. You may or may not be religious. But I give you the following verses that have spoken to me during this journey.

> *(Psalms 103:1-3 NIV)*
>
> **BLESS the LORD, O my soul; And all that is within me, bless His holy name! Bless the LORD, O my soul, and forget not all His benefits. Who forgives all your iniquities, who heals all your diseases?**
>
> *(Deuteronomy 7:15 NIV)*
>
> **And the LORD will take away from you all sickness, and will afflict you with none of the terrible diseases of Egypt, which you have known, but will lay them on all those who hate you.**

(Psalms 30:2 NIV)

O LORD my God, I cried out to You, And You healed me.

(Psalms 34:19 NIV)

Many are the afflictions of the righteous, but the LORD delivers him out of them all.

(Jeremiah 17:14 NIV)

Heal me, O LORD, and I shall be healed; Save me, and I shall be saved, for You are my praise.

Reflection

As I end this journal, it's been 13 months since my first stroke. Many of my deficits still exist. I have good days and bad. Although many of those closest to me understand more, they still don't understand all, so I deal silently with this in my mind. I dream of strokes, hospitals and doctors. I cringe with every headache and bout of heartburn. Each stressful situation brings the same thought to mind, Will this be it? I tell myself it's silly to worry about what we can't control, but we are human. It is in our nature. It is in mine.

So what could be my biggest, most important message to deliver with this book?

It's that no matter what you find yourself facing right now, God knows and understands. He is waiting for you. He is our comforter. He is our healer. He is our friend and our only hope in the good and in the difficult.

I would like to invite you today to accept Jesus Christ as your Savior, if you have never done so. It is really very simple. First you must recognize and Admit that you are a sinner and in need of a savior. Second, you must believe that Jesus is God's son and accept God's free gift of forgiveness and eternal life. Third, you must confess with your mouth your faith in Jesus Christ.

I invite you to pray this simple prayer: Our heavenly Father, forgive me of my sins. I ask you Lord Jesus, who died on the cross for me, to come into my life and become my Savior and Lord. Thank you for your patience in me Lord, and guide me through life from here to eternity. Thank you for loving me God, and for giving me your Son, Jesus Christ. In Jesus name, Amen.

If you have just earnestly prayed that prayer, you now have eternal life in Jesus Christ. There is nothing else for you to do except turn from your sin and live your life for your Savior.

I would encourage you to tell someone that you are a new creation in Jesus Christ. Find a Bible-believing Church or a friend and share your good news with them. Get involved with a group of believers where you can learn and grow. Finally, make sure you realize that being a Christian does not mean you or anyone else is perfect. Instead it means that in Jesus Christ our imperfectness is made complete. I would encourage you to try different Christian churches until you find the one that is right for you and when you do you will know it. It will feel like home, a place where love abounds.

> **"For God so loved the world that He gave his one and only Son, that whoever believes in him shall not perish but have eternal life." (John 3:16 NIV)**

> **"Therefore if any man be in Christ, he is a new creature; Old things are passed away; behold all things are become new." (2 Corinthians 5:17 NIV)**

leave you with this final verse

> **Be strong and courageous. Do not be afraid or terrified, for the Lord your God goes with**

you; he will never leave you nor forsake you."
(Deuteronomy 31:6 NIV)

God is with us my friend. Hold to that. Do not let go. In our darkest hours, he will be there waiting for our call.

God bless you all.

About the Author

Louis Turbeville, currently works in the Oilfield/Instrumentation business as an Account manager, servicing Refineries, Chemical and power plants in the Gulf Coast (Deer Park, Texas) area. Previously, Louis and his wife owned a photography business for 8 years (Action Photos of Texas). Louis studied Instrumentation and Computer Technology at San Jacinto College and University of Houston. He has served San Jacinto Baptist Church in Deer Park for 10 years, serving on the Pastor Leadership team, and as a Trustee. He and his wife Cyndi have been married 19 years, and have three sons, Aaron, Justin and Sean. They also are very proud of their 5 grandchildren, Westin 10, Jaxon 8, Layton 5, Gordon 4 and Cali 2.

Contact Author:
strokeofgod@gmail.com

www.ingramcontent.com/pod-product-compliance
Ingram Content Group UK Ltd.
Pitfield, Milton Keynes, MK11 3LW, UK
UKHW041955230426
12048UKWH00008B/361